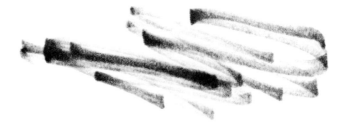

The Alexander Technique

Thorsons First Directions

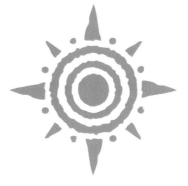

The Alexander Technique

Jeremy Chance

Thorsons
An Imprint of HarperCollins*Publishers*
77-85 Fulham Palace Road,
Hammersmith, London W6 8JB

The Thorsons website address is: www.thorsons.com

Published by Thorsons 2001

Text derived from *Principles of the Alexander Technique*, published by
Thorsons, 1998

10 9 8 7 6 5 4 3 2 1

Editor: Susan Bosanko
Design: Wheelhouse Creative
Production: Melanie Vandevelde
Photography by Henry Allen and PhotoDisc Europe

A catalogue record for this book is available from the British Library

ISBN 0 00711035 9

Printed and bound in Hong Kong

Contents

The Alexander Technique

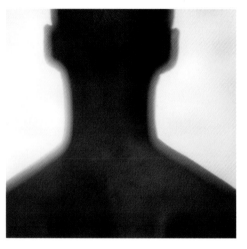

allows release of unnecessary muscle tension

through increased body awareness

What is the Alexander Technique?

Something that makes the Alexander Technique an enigma to everyone who studies it is that you are not going to learn anything new. Everything you will learn you already knew before you started, but you didn't know that you knew it. Confused? Good. You are starting to have your first Alexander experience. Get used to it. In fact, if you try to learn something new you will only hamper your progress. The thing you want to learn is the absence of what you have, and that's nothing.

Alexander's discoveries concern our habits of tension. The primary premise behind Alexander work is that if something is wrong it will be because we are doing something to make it wrong. It's about discovering what we are already doing to our bodies that we don't need to be doing, and then stopping doing it. Then, as Alexander loved to say: 'The right thing does itself.' So Alexander work is about unlearning. It is about increasing an awareness of your body so you can discover, right under your nose, the things you are doing that are causing you unnecessary tension.

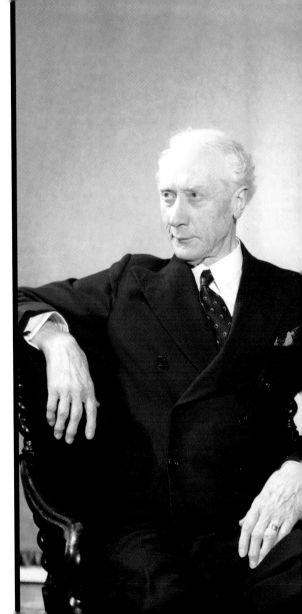

Alexander work is not a therapy or counselling technique, nor is it a treatment, although it can make you feel much, much better. It is a practical technique for changing your reaction to a given stimulus. The criterion upon which a favourable reaction is judged in Alexander work is simply the one that does you less harm, the one that encourages your good health and happiness. You are a pupil, not a patient, and you are going to a lesson. This is very important, because it is easy to confuse this work with therapy for the simple reason that Alexander work definitely does remedy an extraordinary array of ailments.

As well as its practical side, there is an entire conceptual framework within which Alexander work rests. Alexander's own work, as much as anything, is a practical philosophy of life. 'Organised common sense' was one pupil's description. This view is not religious, not even spiritual. It is as practical as Alexander was himself.

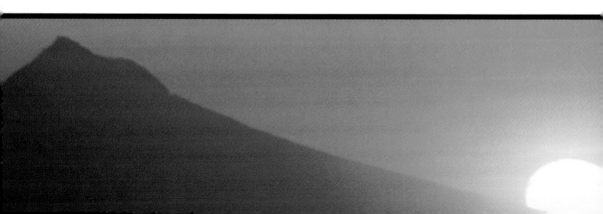

Alexander's Discoveries

F. M. Alexander was beginning to be in demand as an actor in his native Australia, when friendly fellow actors casually mentioned that they could hear him gasping for air during a performance. He was mortified, as he prided himself in avoiding this tiresome habit, so common among the 'declamatory thespians' of his Victorian era. Soon after, he was also getting hoarse.

Resting his voice relieved the hoarseness, but only until his next performance, when it recurred. He concluded that it was something he was doing while performing that caused the problem, and tested this by using mirrors to compare his co-ordination during normal speaking to that during reciting. He was particularly struck by three things: as soon as he started to recite, he tended to pull back his head, depress

his larynx and suck in breath through his mouth to produce a gasping
sound. This was an encouraging discovery. If he did this during reciting
and could manage to stop it, wouldn't his voice then improve?
However, much as he tried, he could not stop this pattern.

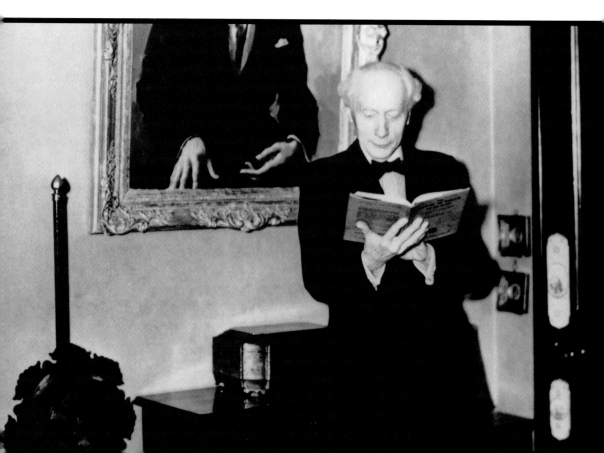

Analysing the problem

Further observation showed him that associated with his head and neck being pulled back, his whole body was collapsing, his shoulders were narrowing and that all the gestures, expressions and actions connected with his performance were intertwined with the movement of his head. He realised that he had been trying to change just a tiny aspect of what was actually a holistically co-ordinated action of all his body parts. There was no one single part of him that needed fixing yet this is how he had been thinking of the problem. He didn't have a voice problem, he was a voice problem. And this meant that he had to change his total reaction before he did anything else.

An empirical thinker, he learnt by watching himself, by thinking about what he saw and then finding an explanation for it, by persevering and practising patiently. He figured out how to co-ordinate his body to achieve some partial relief from his symptoms, confirming that he was on the right track. He slowly came to understand what he needed to do.

He realized that his impulse to move was being driven unconsciously, associated with feelings that had become unreliable. In his mirrors he

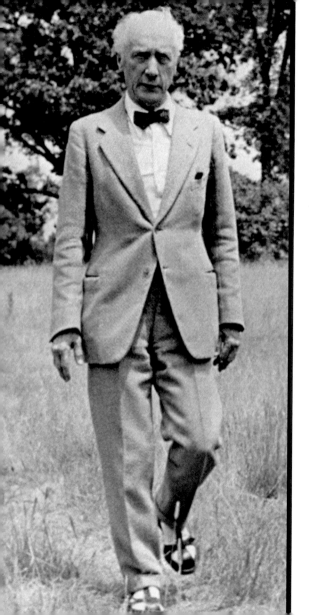

saw that this impulse occurred almost instantaneously in response to the idea of reciting, and the response entailed all the conditions of misuse that he had so meticulously catalogued. It wasn't that one little bit of it occurred and the rest was fine – everything happened and it all happened in one instant. He concluded that if he were ever to be able to react satisfactorily to the stimulus to use his voice, he must replace his old instinctive unreasoned direction of himself by a new conscious direction.

Searching for the answer

He set out to put this idea into practice, but found he still continued with his old habitual response, despite his now more conscious effort to change. What he did next was quite unexpected – he gave up. He decided he just wouldn't try to do the new thing, he would let it go, separate himself completely from the end result he wanted and instead devote his attention to the means. He was telling himself, in effect, that the only way he could gain what he wanted was to stop wanting it. He decided that it was necessary for him to experience the stimulus to speak but to refuse to do anything immediately in response.

This involved long periods of patient silent observation of himself in his mirrors, giving himself directions to change his co-ordination. When he felt that he had practised his means enough and started to use them for the purpose of speaking, he found that he failed more often than he succeeded. He reasoned that the directions he was giving himself were correct, so the problem must lie elsewhere. By careful observation, it dawned on him that his 'feeling' of his directions was disrupting his attempt to change. His feelings were looking for the experience that felt natural, but the experience he actually wanted would feel totally wrong. He was trying to change but simultaneously to stay the same. When he followed his new directions, it felt odd. He had to let go and experience the unfamiliar.

He decided he would make a decision to speak, then give himself the experience of refusing to. At that critical moment, he would give himself his directions and consider his options. Maybe he would speak, maybe he would lift an arm, maybe he would do nothing other than continuing with the process of giving himself directions. He would think, then move, then feel. After he had worked in this way for a considerable time, he became free of his tendency to revert to his wrong habitual use of his body when reciting. After many years of work, he was convinced that at last he was on the right track.

Others observed the remarkable changes in Alexander, and soon people were begging him to teach them his discoveries. He gave up acting, began teaching, continued with his researches, and went on to create the system that today is employed not only by almost every major performing arts institution in the Western world, but also by many thousands of people going about their normal everyday activities and domestic routine.

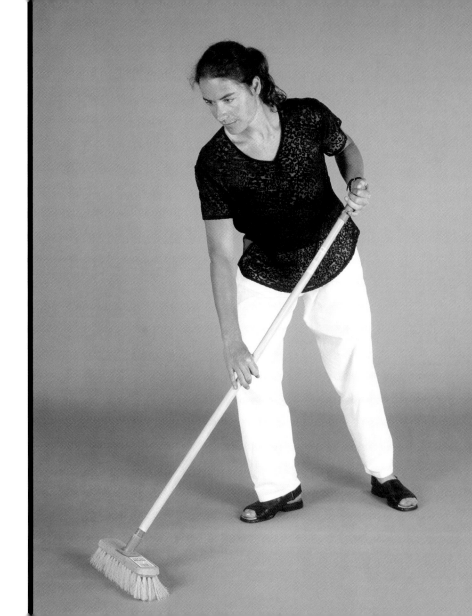

What Can It Do For Me?

The Alexander Technique, before anything else, is a sensation, a new feeling. And what a sensation it is! You come out of your first lesson feeling like you haven't done for years. Your step is light, your neck feels freer and you can sense yourself moving as lithely as a cat. And all your Alexander teacher will have done is rightfully restore a co-ordination that was always yours to begin with.

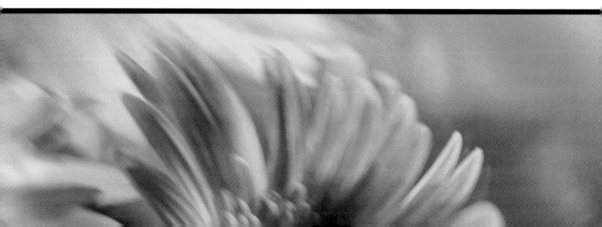

There are three reasons why people undertake Alexander work. First, and by far the most common, is the need to heal: it may be because of a bad back, a repetitive strain injury or just plain stress and tension. Secondly, it may be for professional reasons: musicians, actors, singers, athletes and others pursuing excellence have found the Alexander Technique an invaluable aid to their craft. Thirdly, people come for self-improvement: they are aware that they lack poise, they feel clumsy and awkward with their bodies and want to improve their carriage and sense of confidence.

The list of conditions that have been favourably improved by Alexander lessons is almost embarrassing. These benefits, however, are not the aim of lessons – they are results that arise out of a holistic process. If you practise the Alexander Technique you will be able to make proof of this for yourself. There is also an enormous body of anecdotal evidence from the many hundreds of thousands of people who have experienced such benefits during the century that Alexander's discoveries have been spreading.

Alexander Lessons

Choosing a teacher

Alexander work is very personal and your teacher will learn a great deal about you. You're there to change the habits of a lifetime, so lessons have to go to the essence of your outlook and approach to life. This means it is extremely important for you to find the right teacher.

Not every teacher suits every individual, as there are different styles of Alexander teaching which suit different personalities. Alexander teachers will normally give you a first lesson with no further commitment, so providing the opportunity to discuss your situation, determine costs, frequency and overall number of lessons, as well as any anticipated results. You will also have the chance to assess whether you feel comfortable with the teacher and their work. How a teacher affects you depends on their skill, your receptivity as a student and the chemistry of both your personalities.

Alexander work is an educational process so you should learn something, even in your first lesson. Your teacher should have the skill to get this 'something' across to you and not leave you completely mystified.

The success of Alexander work is in direct ratio to your own receptivity to it. A good Alexander teacher uses their hands to stimulate your nervous system to respond in a particular way. For that to succeed, you need to co-operate. Alexander work is so subtle that some people at first think nothing is happening. If you're cynical, looking for fault and wanting to gain evidence for a negative outcome, you will probably find it. Motivation is everything.

Make sure the chemistry with your teacher works for you. If it does, your experiences will deepen with each lesson. If not, you will always be protecting a little bit of yourself, and this protection is nothing else but a kind of tension. Alexander lessons aren't like anything else so it's important to get the right teacher before you commit yourself and begin regular lessons.

Using touch

Your teacher will touch you, continuously, using their hands to listen, to invite and to tell. You remain fully clothed throughout the lesson.

Alexander teachers are trained to listen to your body with their hands, using them to pick up an incredible amount of information about the continuously occurring subtle shifts of balance in your co-ordination. Having understood the pattern of co-ordination you are currently making, teachers then use their hands to talk to your nervous system directly and invite it to make a different kind of inner dance, one that doesn't cause so much pressure and tension in your body. This can be quite a complex invitation. Then, when a teacher's hands are really effective, they do tell your co-ordination what to do. You watch the results in amazement as your body transforms without you seeming to do anything.

During the lesson

A lesson can proceed in many different ways. Every lesson has one purpose of offering you a new sensation of co-ordinating yourself in an initially unfamiliar but easier and more natural manner. More importantly, each lesson seeks to put that new sensation into a context that you can understand. You are there to learn how to generate this sensation for yourself. This is achieved through a delicate interplay between the processes of observation, interpretation and experimentation. These three processes are applied to chairwork, tablework and activities.

There will most probably be three things in the teaching room: a chair, a table and a mirror. The chair is for chairwork, the table for tablework and the mirror is for you to see that, as the lesson progresses, you don't actually look at all like the way you feel you must be looking.

Chairwork

This is the classic activity around which most Alexander teachers centre their lessons. It involves you getting in and out of a chair with the teacher's assistance and each time gives rise to a new result. You

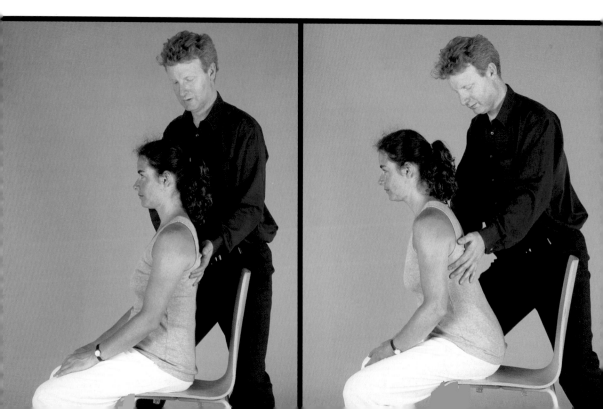

are not actually learning how to get out of a chair – this is a device, a method, not an end in itself. It is a technique used in order to bring about a condition of co-ordination that is more beneficial to you. Once you have learnt this procedure, you can apply it anywhere, at anytime and to anything.

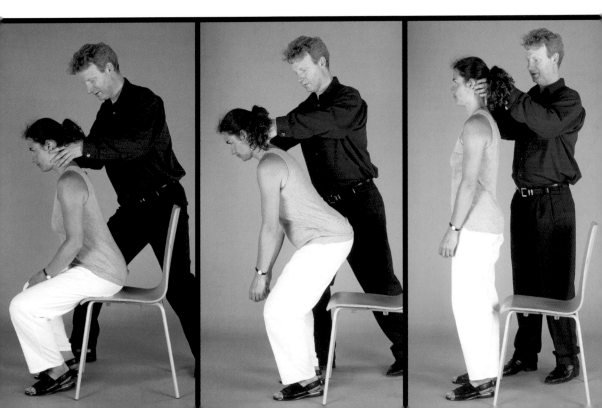

Tablework

In tablework you lie down on your back in semi-supine position (with your knees bent up and your head resting on some books) while the teacher gently helps to lengthen your torso, arms and legs. Some teachers will work on you silently, others will chat away about anything. Some will give you guided instructions as to what to think and still others will ask you to actively participate in different procedures and activities, all as you remain lying on your back.

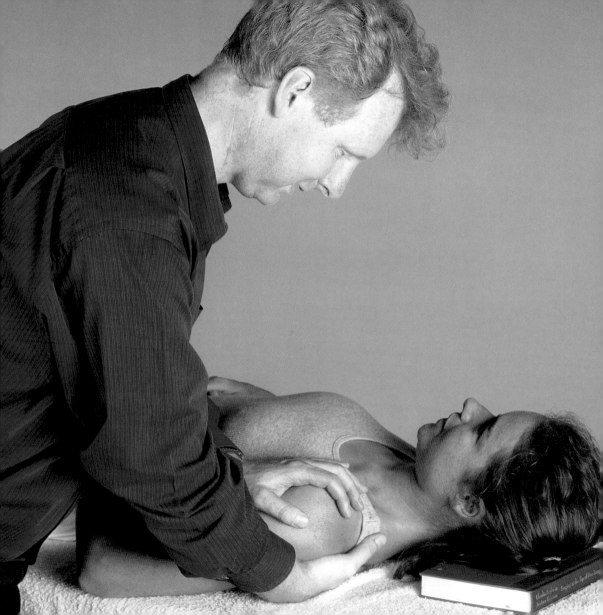

Activities

Chairwork is an activity but aside from that, most teachers will at least explore walking, bending and doing things with your arms. Remember, it is the principles being used to change your co-ordination that are the focus of learning, not the activity itself, so ultimately it doesn't matter what activity you do.

That said, it is often of value to explore Alexander's discoveries in relation to any specialized activities that you are involved in regularly as part of your daily life. If you examine them in your lesson, the activity itself will serve as a reminder to apply what you are learning.

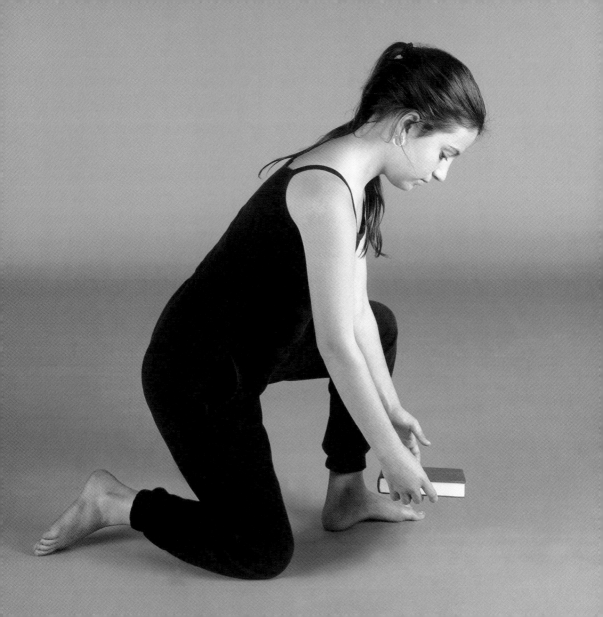

Many Alexander teachers have another professional skill, as musicians, actors, athletes, martial arts practitioners, etc. It makes sense to go to a teacher who understands the demands of your particular profession or chosen form of recreational activity, so it's worth enquiring about a teacher's background, especially when faced with a choice.

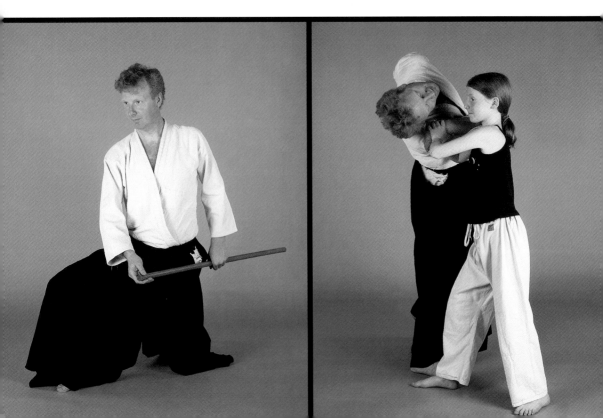

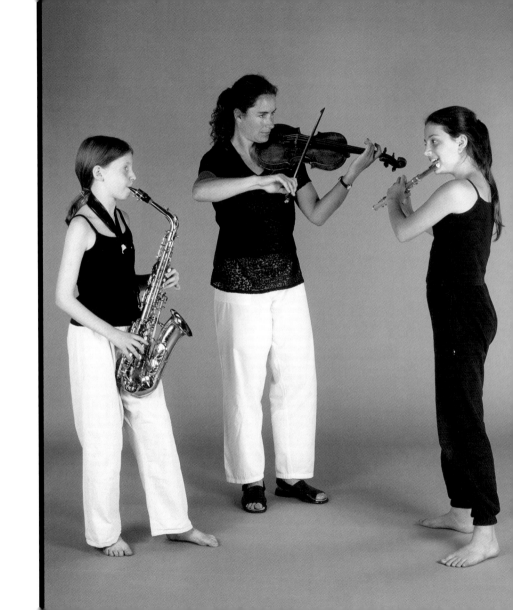

What have you learned?

A lesson is about changing the state of your consciousness and, as such, is best understood through experience alone. Lessons teach you how to keep applying the three processes – observation, interpretation and experimentation – in order to gain this experience, regardless of the type of activity you are doing. While there are many different activities you can explore in your lessons, there are no set exercises that you can go home and show others or practise on your own.

The effect of lessons tends to build exponentially, week by week. It is a good idea to keep a journal, as progress can seem slow until you look back and realize how much has changed. In Alexander lessons you are always intrigued by the next problem so it is sometimes too easy to forget just how far along you have actually progressed. A journal will help to keep your perspective on the process.

Alexander lessons will open you up to an entire new domain of knowledge about yourself, a new universe of experience that beckons to be understood. As this world reveals itself to you there can be amazing and unexpected results.

Working on Yourself Alone

These suggestions for working on your own aim for the same result as a traditional Alexander lesson. However, a lesson has the primary ingredient of 'sensation' facilitated by the hands of your teacher, an ingredient that is missing when you work on your own.

Some Alexander teachers feel that working alone is inappropriate, mainly because they are concerned that you will confuse or even harm yourself, and they have a point. The easiest way to understand the Alexander Technique is to take lessons, and then you will find the information given here a useful aid to understanding. So there is no guarantee that you won't cause yourself problems, but if you cannot get to a teacher then these procedures can, if followed carefully, guide you to generate a different quality of co-ordination.

These experiments require discipline, a lot of patience, time, and a willingness to experience confusion, frustration and failure. It is by no means certain that these procedures will bring any immediate benefit, it depends on your ability to understand and apply them. Like everything worthwhile, it takes practise, but if you persevere, the light will come on. To help you practise, I have also produced a tape, *Principles of the Alexander Technique*, available from the publisher.

Primary control

The head leads and the body follows. In everything. Alexander once called it 'the true and primary movement'. Now it goes by the name 'primary control' and a simple activity will allow you to experience it. Get down on all fours and have a friend gently take your head within their hands as shown in the illustration. Now let your friend guide you by delicately turning your head to look left or right. You will experience that you are impelled to crawl in the direction that your head is being

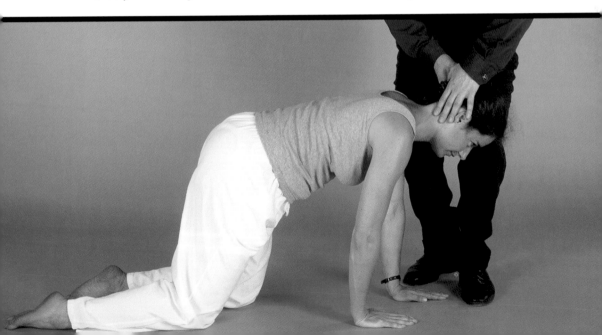

led. Try not to go that way: leave your head free to be led by your partner, but at the same time attempt to crawl in the opposite direction. It's near impossible, unless you can turn your head that way too. The head leads and the body follows.

The relationship of your head/neck to your body is always influencing your co-ordination, sometimes beneficially, more often than not harmfully. If you get neck tension, a sore back, sore knees, breathing difficulties, or unnecessary tension of any kind, you are probably pulling your head back and down, as shown here, and shortening your body.

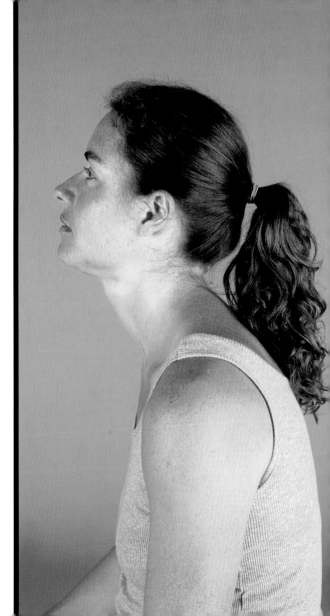

Proprioception

Proprioception is the body's ability to sense itself, and it is vital that you first train yourself in the use of your proprioceptive sense, learning to utilize this powerful imaging system hardwired into your nervous system.

Millions of proprioceptive receptors are located in every muscle, ligament and tendon of your body. These receptors are firing off their messages continuously, but we largely suppress awareness of this input in favour of our other senses, all of which are concerned with determining our relationship with phenomena external to us. Only one sense deals entirely with our internal universe: the proprioceptive sense. It is a miracle sense which, if accessed fully, has a wealth of previously unrealized information about ourselves. The more you practise using it, the more natural it becomes to be mindful of your body and have an accurate awareness of your co-ordination. This benefit will eventually extend to activities such as walking, bending and all the other things you do in a day.

Remaining still

Exploring your proprioceptive sense requires that you remain still for a period of time. You decide how long, but 10 minutes is sufficient to start.

Why is it that so many people dread the idea of staying still? Why do we fidget and wiggle about all the time? Watch yourself right now. Are you remaining quietly still as you read or are you shaking your foot, fiddling with your hair, chewing gum, biting your lip, holding your legs unnecessarily tight or grabbing on with something else? If you observe yourself carefully you will find that you are doing something which, upon honest analysis, isn't really necessary. Stop these activities. Just remain still and quietly watch yourself. Try it now as you read. Can you do it? For how long?

A primary motivation for all this fidgeting is that we are attempting to get away from ourselves, away from some feeling of discomfort or agitation. Analyse a few of your fidgeting actions. Why do you do them? What is the impulse, the need, that the fidgeting answers within you? Is it a seeking, a wanting-of-something, directing each movement? Check it out.

Making adjustments and movements all of the time does serve to distract us from experiencing our underlying condition. When we do stop and experience that condition, it can be quite overwhelming within a few seconds. Dizziness, nausea, fear, nervousness and irritation are not uncommon initial experiences. For a lucky few, it feels blissful, a relief to stop in this way. Your experience will probably fall somewhere between these two extremes.

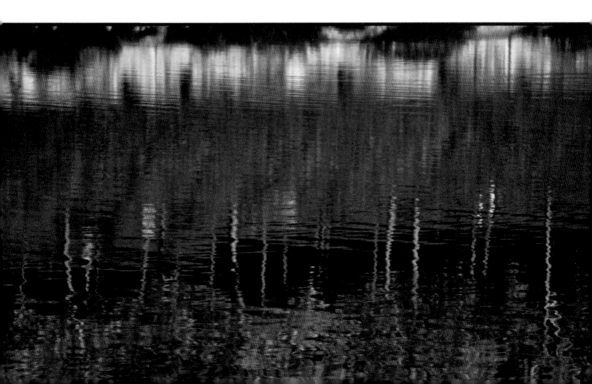

Self-acceptance

There is a deeper meaning to this step of becoming still, and that is to accept yourself. Be comfortable with being uncomfortable. Give up trying to make things better. Embrace yourself with all your imperfections. It isn't possible to make changes against a background of denial. Denial, in this case, means trying not to be who you are being.

Most of your postural adjustments are most likely made against a background of wanting to get rid of some discomfort. It is as though you are using the discomfort to push yourself somewhere else, and there's the irony. In order to push you need something to push on, so no matter how hard you try to get away from your discomfort, you always need it to do the getting away, so it always goes with you. It's a Catch-22 situation.

Self-acceptance is paradoxically a way of escaping from this never-ending cycle. You learn to stop seeing yourself as a mistake waiting to be fixed and move deeper into your feelings of discomfort. Instead of fighting yourself, you start to tolerate yourself, even feel love and compassion towards yourself.

During the first minutes of remaining quiet, the urges to move don't stop. Observe them with indifference, each time freshly making a decision: 'No, I won't make that movement, I will continue to remain quiet and still within my body and accept these conditions as they are.' If you keep working on this premise of accepting yourself, a strange thing evolves out of it: it becomes easier, almost pleasurable, to remain this way. When your mind has quieted to the point where you no longer feel urges to keep adjusting some part of your body, then you are ready to move on.

In the beginning you may never get beyond this first step. That's fine, as it is better to take the time to calm your mind than to proceed in an agitated state. Proceeding in that way is entirely contrary to the whole process.

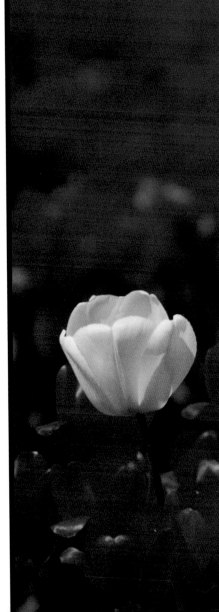

Working seated

Mapping your primary holding pattern

This step involves sensing the primary holding pattern of your musculature, the pattern formed by the deep, intrinsic 'being' muscles that maintain your integrity during movement. It is your personality's signature and a reservoir of unexpressed emotion. Expect to occasionally experience strong emotions as you continue practising this procedure.

You don't begin with emotions, however, you begin practically by slowly mapping out the relative spatial relationships between different parts of your body. I will guide you through mapping yourself while sitting in a chair, as it is a common everyday activity. However, as you develop this practice it is good to explore all kinds of different orientations. Take a sitting position that you consider comfortable rather than trying to sit correctly. When you have achieved a degree of quiet, begin mapping your body.

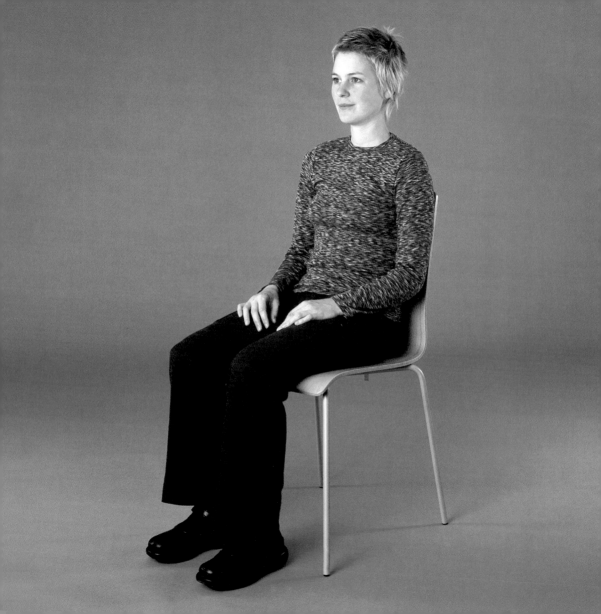

Your shoulder-arms

Arms don't end at the shoulder because your shoulder is just part of
your arm. If you were a bird the arm part would have all the feathers
on it, whereas the shoulder part is where all the muscle power and
movement of the arm is anchored. To get around the division that
language makes, we can call it the shoulder-arm.

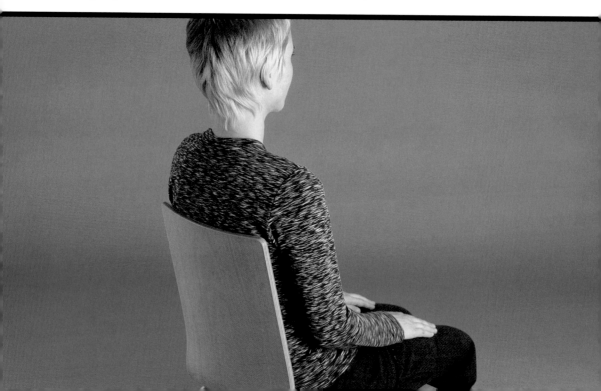

Compare your two shoulder-arms. Which is tighter? If you are not sure, just leave your attention on them both and wait. A stronger impression will emerge. The waiting gives you time to discern the subtle proprioceptive feedback that is coming from these two shoulder-arms (part of this practice concerns developing greater sensitivity to proprioceptive feedback). Ask yourself if your shoulder-arms feel exactly the same. This is next to impossible. Then contemplate how they are different. Keep creatively sensing them both – the top, the bottom, the inside and the outside of everything you consider to be a 'shoulder' and an 'arm'.

Now begin orientating their position in space relative to each other. Which is higher? Which is further forward? Again, wait until a definite impression emerges. Often it won't become immediately apparent, but, after time, you will gain a clearer impression. You may have felt that you started in a straight position, but as you go in you might feel you are twisted around. Once you have a clear impression, move on.

Your head and neck

Just where does your shoulder-arm end and your neck begin? Of course this is an impossible question because there is no such place. So widen the sense of your shoulder-arms to include the two sides of your neck. It is important in this process of mapping your holding pattern that you build upon the previous mapping you have done. In this case, retain the impression of your shoulder-arms as you expand your area of awareness to include mapping your head and neck.

Which side of your neck is tighter? Does this relate to your shoulder-arm that feels tighter – can you feel how this tension is continuous throughout the whole area? As with the shoulder-arm, transform this feeling of tension into a spatial orientation: which side of the neck feels shorter? Are you leaning your head more to one side? How does this fit in with what you are experiencing with your shoulder-arms? Again, take time until a clear impression of your shoulder-arms and head leaning emerges. Spend as much time as it takes to get to this point. Don't go on until you have a clear inner image of these areas.

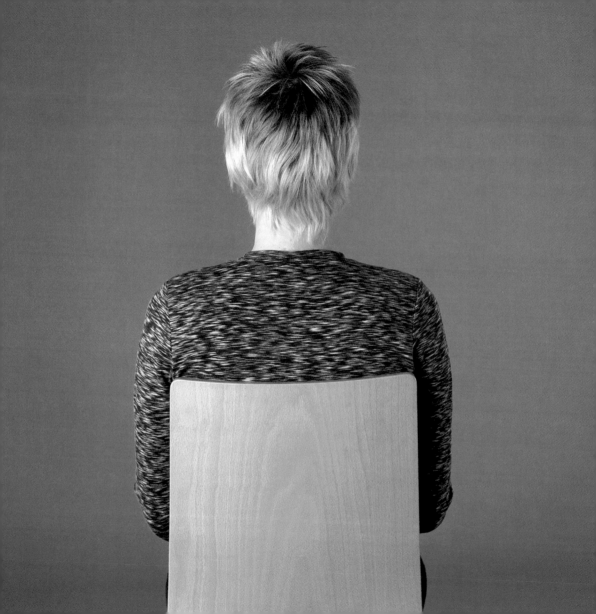

Your rib cage and pelvis

Now sense the contact of your back against the chair. While you maintain the awareness of your shoulder-arms, neck and head, check which side of your back has more contact or pressure against the back of the chair. Are you making contact with the back of the chair with the same or different areas of your back? Can you relate that back to your shoulder-arms and head and neck and make sense of it as part of a whole pattern of holding?

Check the two sides of your rib cage between the bottom ribs and the top of the pelvic bone on the two sides of your body. Do these two sides feel as long as each other, or does it feel as if one side is shorter because your rib cage is compressed down more on one side? Again, relate this back to everything else you are sensing and discover how this all fits together into a pattern of holding. Don't go on to the next step until you succeed in generating this new awareness. Keep practising until you do.

Now sense the contact your sitting bones have with the chair. Are you right on them or sitting on the back part of your bottom? Is the pressure equal on both sides or can you feel more on one side than the other? How does this follow from what is happening in the rest of your body? How is it fitting into an overall pattern of holding?

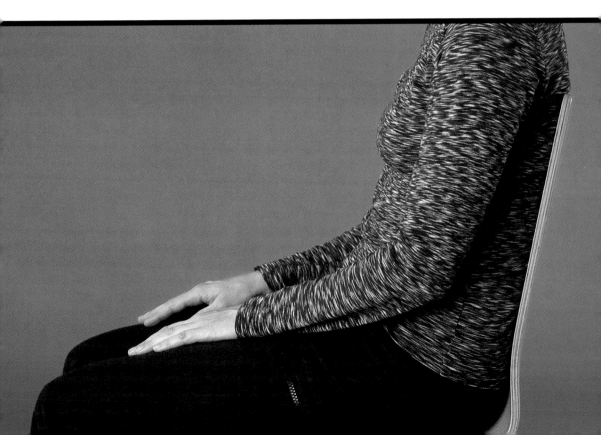

Your legs, knees and feet

While still enlivening the overall map of your body generated up to now expand it into an awareness of both your legs. Particularly sense the position of your knees relative to each other. Is one pulled in more than the other? Alternatively, does one feel more spread out than the other? Can you feel how this is a result of the whole primary holding pattern throughout your body? That the position of your head, shoulder-arms, rib cage and pelvis all combine to cause your two legs to be in the position they are in?

Finally, with this overall awareness, check out your feet and how they are placed on the floor (if indeed they are both on the floor). Which part of your foot has more pressure on it? Are you collapsing the foot inwards into the arch or turning it outwards and lifting the arch off the floor? Can you understand this movement relative to the position of your knees and the body above it? Figure out how it fits in with the whole pattern from head down. With practice this whole stage can be done in as little as a few seconds or even less. Remember, the information is always there – learning to listen and interpret it is all you're practising to do.

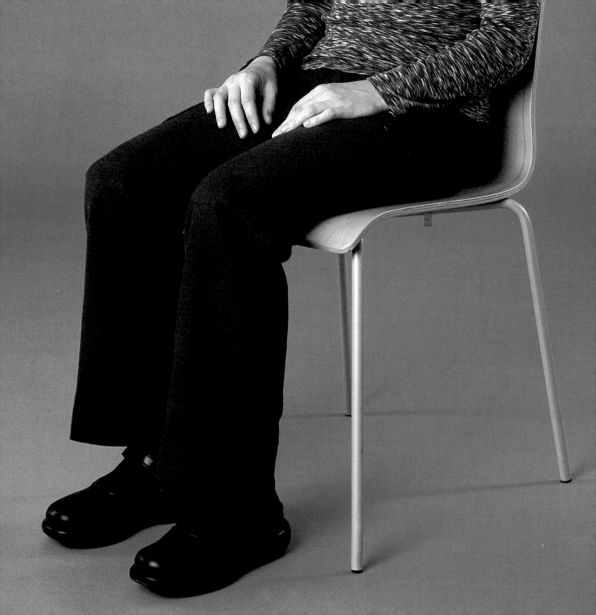

Making the parts whole

By now it has become clearer that you are twisting your body a little to the left or the right (this is almost universally true). Keep up the questions, thinking up your own and being creative about it, until a clear impression of a whole body twist begins to emerge. If initially you can't discern a twist, keep up the questions and your patience until an impression finally emerges. It always does.

Often it arrives in a sudden flash. This is the point you were working towards, to realize that you are holding yourself in an overall twist from the top of your head to the tip of your feet.

There are hundreds of different ways you can go about mapping this pattern, and it is for you to take this blueprint and start to work creatively on your own. However, it is important that your impression of this overall holding pattern arises by itself, that it isn't an intellectual imposition on your body arising from abstract notions you may currently entertain or according to what some expert told you. Even if the expert is right you still have to experience it within yourself. Truly understanding is feeling, not just a dry, intellectual knowing. If done correctly, this procedure definitely gives you the feeling of discovering something that was there all the time but hidden from your awareness. It is important not to think you know already what you are doing before you start, even if you have practised this process a hundred times.

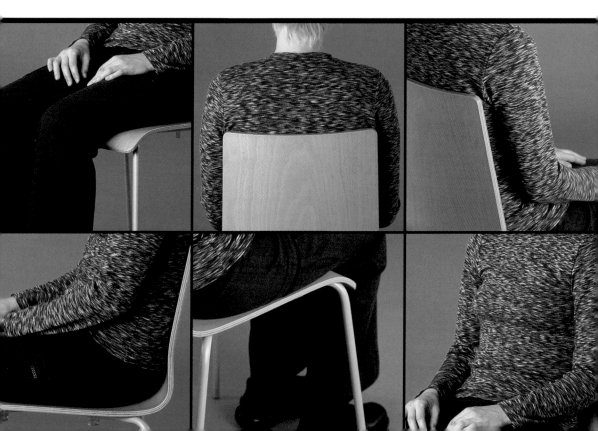

Going in further

Having gained this holistic awareness of your primary holding pattern, it is time to play with it a little, to develop your relationship to this pattern. There are several alternative strategies to take. You can try them out one after the other, or each one alone during any one session.

First, remain sensing the holding pattern in a non-linear way. Previously you built up an impression step-by-step, moving through your body from the top down. Your attention has been deliberately directed along certain lines. Now, let your attention be free to roam where it wants to. This still means focusing on the body, not drifting off into unrelated day-dreaming, but there is no order to it, no logic in it. This can deepen your perception of your whole holding pattern, revealing previously unrecognized aspects of it. Be intuitive, go with what suggests itself.

Secondly, it is useful to accentuate the holding pattern. Twist more in the direction you feel you are already going in. Do this very delicately, with great awareness of the whole pattern throughout the process of exaggerating it. Determine where you make the effort, which muscle groups seem to be engaged to exaggerate your holding. Does the exaggerated movement increase the strain you feel at different places in your body? Where? Can you feel if it starts in a particular place or does it happen as a whole? Is more work done in one place compared to another?

Thirdly, experience the emotional charge of your holding pattern. Feel it as an attitude, a way you have of relating to the world, a communication you are making to others about yourself. Are you accepting, fighting or withdrawing from the world? Or are you pulling away with one part, pushing against with another? Do you feel weak or strong? Is there a sadness set within you, or frustration and irritation, even anger?

Simply let these impressions emerge of their own accord. The act of focusing attention is enough. If nothing emerges, don't force it. Revisit the process another time.

Undoing

Our usual attempts to correct a feeling of tension and discomfort involve us going against the tension spot, as in making an effort to sit up against the tendency to slump. Instead we are going into our tension, embracing it, coming to know it intimately and, through that process, letting the holding pattern simply dissolve away and undo itself.

If you have followed the previous steps carefully, this step actually needs no explanation. Once you fully realize the extent of your holding pattern, the undoing does itself. It's as though you wake up to all the holding you are doing and, because you sense it so clearly, there is nothing to figure out any more and releasing it is obvious. If you can't release easily it is axiomatic that you haven't seen your pattern clearly and you need to repeat the earlier steps more thoroughly.

As you release your holding pattern, expect it to feel strange, even wrong. Also expect suddenly to release the aches and tension you feel. If you don't experience that, you are being too forceful. This is the key moment. If you have done well, and move delicately, now's the time you get results. It is a sweet moment and worth all the effort, because this experience can stay with you for days.

Introducing movement

Being simplistic we could say that up until now you have only investigated the intrinsic, muscular holding pattern of the being muscles. Although it is vital, it isn't the whole story. Interlaced and layered over this holding pattern, and interacting with and affecting it, are the larger 'doing' muscle groups that are responsible for the bigger movements of walking, bending, using the arms and legs, etc. How do these bigger movements affect your primary holding pattern and how does your primary holding pattern affect these bigger movements?

A simple movement to pick for answering these questions is to move forward in the chair. Sit back in the chair and go through all the previous steps, up to and including the release of your primary holding pattern. At this time consider the idea of moving forward. Immediately you think that thought, observe the result in your body. Research has shown that merely the thought of a movement causes activity in the muscles that will eventually perform it. Your aim is to reach a degree of sensitivity so that you can detect these subtle changes before you actually move. At the very moment you detect yourself tensing, release out of the decision to move and go back to just sitting again.

Spend a lot of time dancing between these two movements (beginning to move forward in the chair and subsequently releasing by deciding against this action). The decision to move and the decision to stop have to be genuine, and not a ruse for observation. As you observe this dance around the critical moment of action/non-action, you can analyse all the preparatory movements you make to move forward from the chair.

How do these preparatory movements compare to your habitual primary holding pattern? Do you feel yourself going back into the pulls and tightening that you just spent time thinking yourself out of? This step is another useful way of giving you an impression of your primary holding pattern. Using this step and the previous ones you can explore it thoroughly, first in stillness, then in activity.

Can you move forward in the chair without going back into your habitual holding pattern? It should feel very strange even to attempt to do this. Your feelings, being unfamiliar with this kind of co-ordination, will balk at any attempt to move this way. There will be an overwhelming feeling that you have to pull down in the way you are accustomed to in order to move forward in the chair. Check it out. Have you pulled back into your habitual holding pattern at all?

Did the moving forward from the chair feel easier than usual or did it feel stiff?

You have to be very honest with yourself at this point. We all love to succeed but the truth is you are most likely to have failed. The failure is in fact the basis of success, of learning. Expect it, embrace it, reconsider what you have done and experiment again. The most common fault at this time is to brace and stiffen yourself by trying to hold yourself in a new position while you move forward from the chair. Don't be discouraged, as this happens all the time. Be patient and kind with yourself, and keep experimenting. This is a long-term process, not a quick fix.

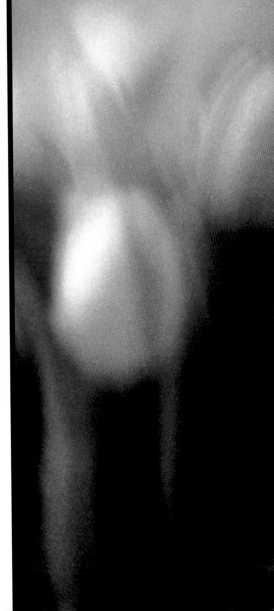

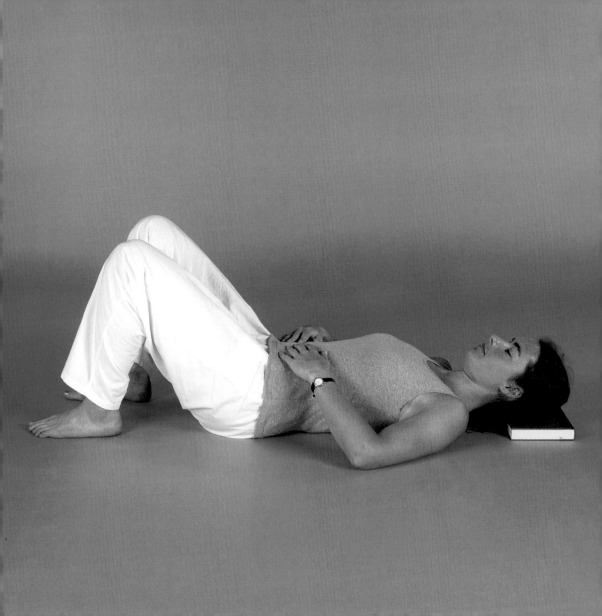

Working in semi-supine

Semi-supine position

This position engineers your spine to be at maximum rest, allowing its curves to lengthen and assisting a releasing of the intrinsic 'being' muscles of your spine that are mostly in an unnecessarily tight and contracted state. The intervertebral discs of your spine, which act as shock absorbers and which are under considerable pressure while you are upright, have a chance to rejuvenate themselves. Semi-supine also offers you an opportunity to explore your holding pattern and its release while in a passive and undemanding position of co-ordination. It beats slumping in a chair when you get home. Alexander teachers call it constructive rest.

Getting into semi-supine

Place a book on the floor, stand a half-body's distance from it, and follow the procedure shown in the illustrations to get down into position. It is worthwhile getting down into semi-supine thoughtfully. Taking time to arrive in the position with a little length is vastly superior to getting down hurriedly and ending up contracted, twisted and generally shortened through your body.

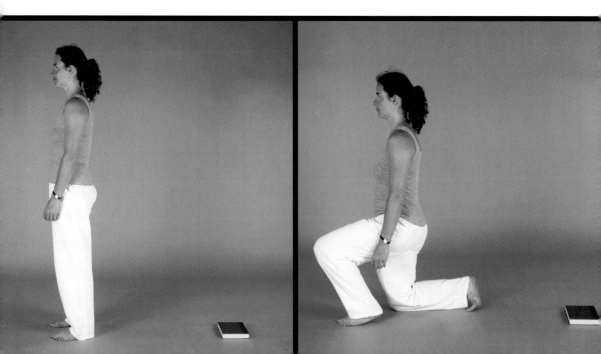

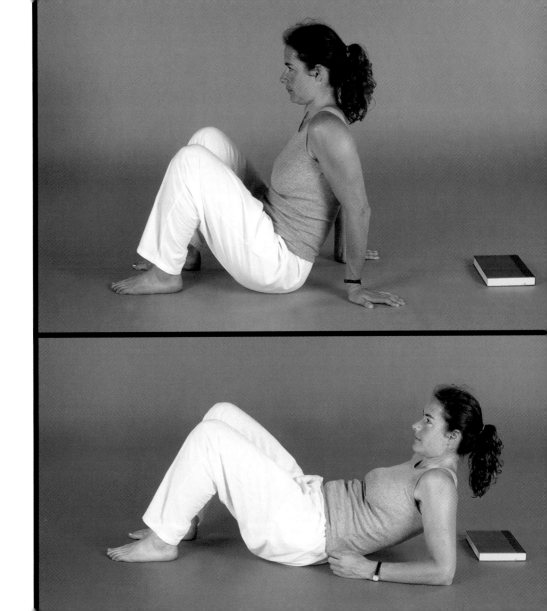

Experiment with different heights of book until you find one that feels neither too high (tucking your chin in too close to your neck) nor too low (feeling that your head is falling back) but seems comfortable for you. The aim is to bring your head to a height that leaves it in as neutral a relation to the rest of the spine as it would be when standing and looking straight ahead. Use books, not a cushion, because books give your head a firm contact, stopping it from sinking backwards. If your head presses too hard and feels uncomfortable, use a towel to soften the contact, but still make sure it is a firm surface. Your neck should be free of any contact with the books.

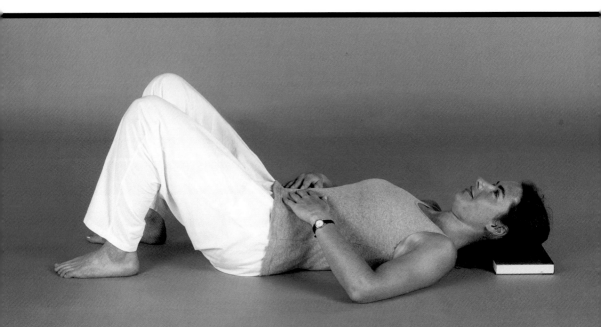

Your knees are bent up to take pressure off your lower back. If you find it difficult to keep your legs up (some people find they keep falling outwards) you could place some large cushions under each knee and rest your legs on them. Some people place a chair underneath the lower half of their legs, but that will only work if the chair is roughly equal to the height of your knees.

Check your lower back. Is it in contact with the floor or is there still an arch? If there is, avoid lifting your pelvis and tucking in your bottom to flatten it out against the floor. Instead get down again, this time checking that you don't arch your back in as you unroll your torso down onto the floor. If there is still an arch, leave it. With time and practice this arch will usually level to make contact with the floor.

Your arms are best placed on your torso where they feel easy and comfortable. For some people this may mean on your hips, for others on your tummy. Experiment a little to find out what seems natural. Don't hold your hands together, as it is better that they don't touch. This assists you in becoming aware of each separately and avoids creating unnecessary tension. Alternatively, you can place your hands beside your body rather than on it, with your palms facing down to the floor roughly at the level of your lower back.

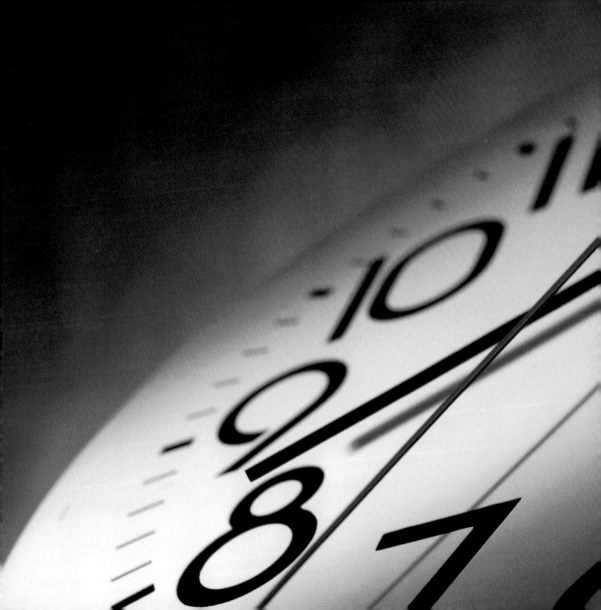

Mapping and releasing

Listen, sense and observe your body before projecting any messages to release it. Take the time to get to know your tension well. Become its friend and then you'll be able to understand it. Start by simply being with yourself. Just being, not trying to fix, make better, correct or adjust anything. Open the space of your body by giving time for your thoughts. Quit the feeling of being in a hurry. Instead, give yourself time, lots and lots of time, and let the process unfold at its own pace without you trying to force things along. Become aware of all the subtle vibrations and movements that are happening continuously throughout your body. Just being with the sensations as they arise is enough – this by itself leads you to understand what will be useful to 'direct' into your body when it comes time to do that.

When you have achieved a degree of quiet, begin mapping your body, exploring your holding pattern and allowing it to release as you did when sitting in a chair. When in semi-supine it is generally good to begin with your head and neck, then progress down your torso (ribs and pelvis) and arms (shoulders, elbows and hands) and finally to the legs (hips, knees and feet).

By collecting together the awareness of several areas all together, one after the other, there is a greater chance that you will magically hit upon a pattern of holding of which you had previously been unaware. By understanding the holistic operation of your co-ordination, you have a better chance of unmasking and releasing the patterns that create unnecessary tension.

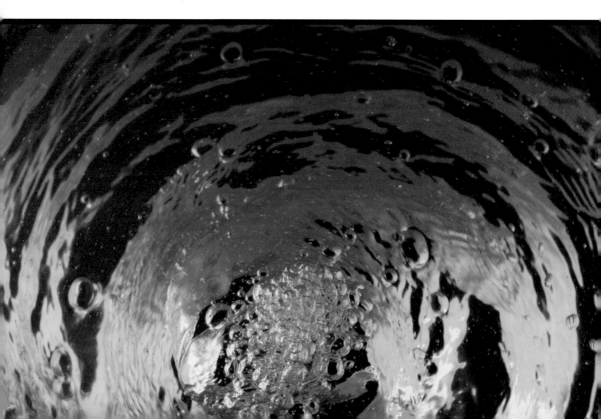

Working standing with mirrors

These experiments are along the lines that Alexander himself followed. First, as Alexander did, get yourself at least two mirrors and position them at an angle to each other, as shown on page 72, so you can easily see your profile without having to twist your neck.

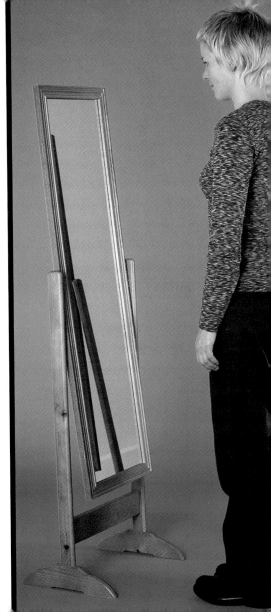

Preliminary stance

All these experiments are done while standing, so you need to consider your preliminary stance. You probably have many ideas about correct and incorrect posture and you might even try to put these into effect by standing up straight or holding yourself more erect.

Slouching and standing up straight are not separate: they are two sides of the same thing, and always exist together. If you want to rid yourself of your slouch, just standing up straight won't work. So don't bother trying to correct your posture in any way. Just let yourself be as you find yourself. You may not like how you feel or look, but it's the truth. Accept it, and just assume your normal everyday posture.

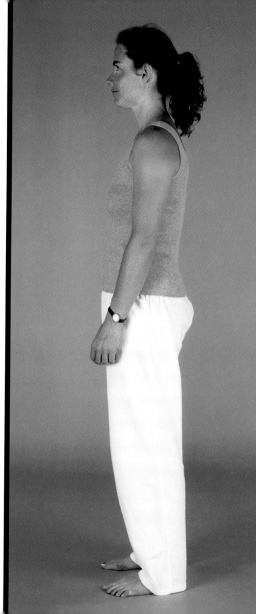

Your aim

As with the seated and semi-supine experiments and procedures, you are going to explore your holding pattern and through such discovery, allow it to release. Use what you have already discovered in these other positions while you work standing. Remember, you are experimenting, so do not expect anything, and be careful not to find what you think you should be looking for. Instead find what is actually happening.

Specifically, you are going to discover how to allow your neck to be free in such a way that your head can go forwards and up and your body can lengthen.

A free neck

Think of your mind or thoughts as part of your body's movements: your thoughts are how your muscles behave. So letting your neck be free isn't something you can do, for it is the result of your not doing something. Similarly with lengthening. All a muscle can do is contract. Lengthening results when a muscle stops contracting.

In Alexander work a free neck is one that allows your head to go forwards and up. It is dynamic, alert and poised. A free neck doesn't mean one without tension, or just letting your head flop around like a rag doll. There has to be tension, or your head would nod off as it does when you're sleepy.

The real question is: how much tension? And the answer is: enough that your head isn't pulled back and down, which means, by inference, that it must be going forwards and up. To discover forwards and up, you first need to experience the opposite, which is backwards and down.

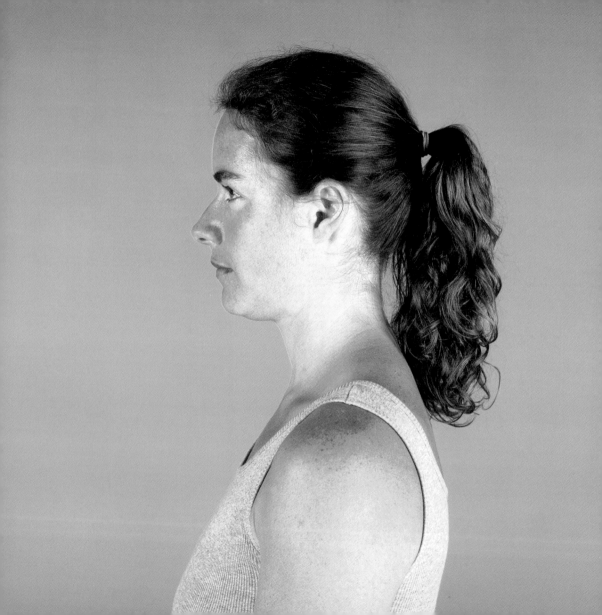

Tilting your head

Tilt *only* your head forwards. Did you also bend your neck forward, as shown in the picture? In 99% of cases the answer is yes, despite the fact that you were asked to tilt *only* your head. What does this prove? That most people think of their neck and head as one unit, not as separate elements that combine to make movements. Actually, the top joint of the spine is at the level of your earlobes.

Now tilt your head forwards again, watching that the only movement is at that head/neck joint. You'll discover that the movement is tiny, almost negligible. If it feels big to you, look in your mirrors and check whether you're bending your neck forwards as well.

Having discovered this difference between your head and neck, you can now explore further.

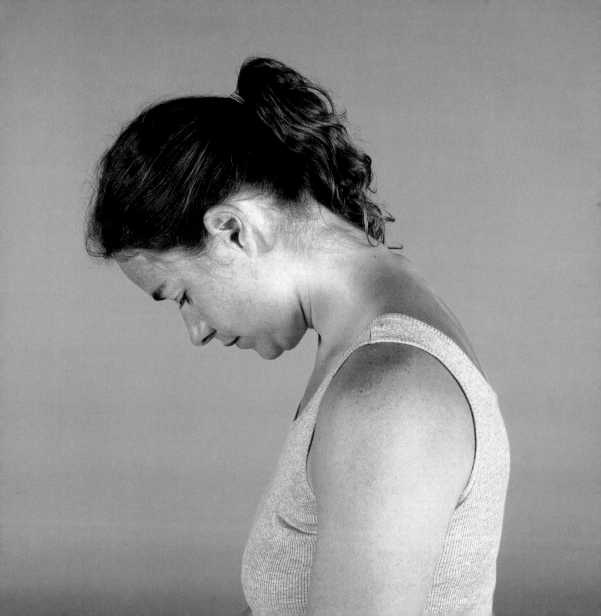

Discovering backwards and down

Begin by just looking. Is your head moving? At first you might think it isn't, but you're wrong, it is. Look again more carefully. Be patient and keep watching until, eventually, you can see that it is. Now you are ready to begin observing your movements.

Say something and watch where your head moves. Do this at least 20 or 30 times, until you are sure you can see yourself doing almost the same thing every time you speak. There will be other things you are doing that are slightly different every time, but there will be one thing that is constant. Can you figure out what it is?

Continue watching yourself, but now shout something. Do this many times. What do your head and neck do? Start comparing yourself speaking and shouting (again many times), asking yourself if they are different. They will be, but how are they different? How do you move your head and neck each time?

Persevere with these experiments patiently until you figure out what you are doing with your head and neck. Most of you will observe that

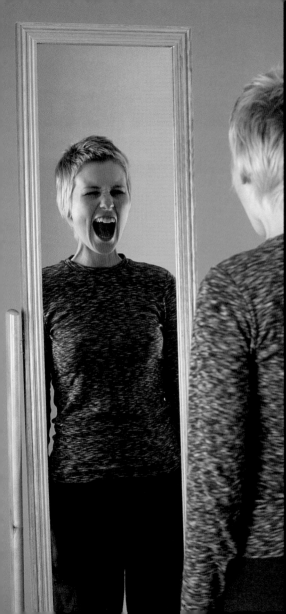

you pull your head back, lifting your chin up, while also dropping your neck down to create a combined effect of head back and neck down. Take plenty of time to watch and learn how you co-ordinate yourself. Work until you are crystal clear about the movements of your head and neck.

You also need to explore the flow-on effect that these movements have on the remainder of your co-ordination, as what your neck does is connected with the movement of your whole torso. For example, to compensate for bending your neck down, you will probably arch your torso back from the lower back, which in turn increases the inward curve at your lower back and results in thrusting your hips forward.

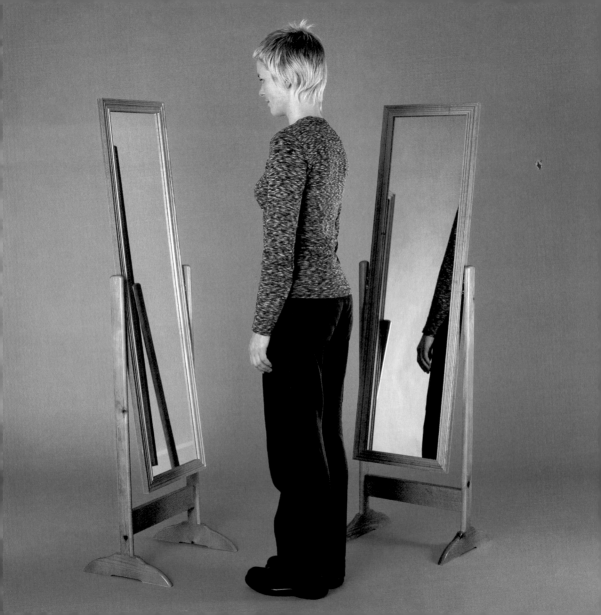

Discovering shortening

Resume your preliminary stance in front of your mirrors. Again start by just looking. The temptation is to start correcting things by readjusting your stance, but resist doing that. Be still and watch. As you watch you will notice that you can't be completely still, it's impossible. Very subtly you are rocking back and forth and around in a circle on your two feet.

Watch that carefully for a long time, seeing if you can discern any pattern to that movement. Is it connected with your breathing at all? It may be or it may be not – that's for you to figure out. Analyse the movement carefully. Where does it occur most? How does it affect the balance of your head and neck?

Rib and torso movements

Watch the movement of your whole rib cage. You will perhaps see that while your rib cage slumps down, your whole upper torso manages to arch back from the lower back. Check if your head is going back and your neck going down. If so, can you feel that the downward compression of your rib cage results from the pressure that having your neck down places on it? When you rock back, does your upper torso move backwards in space by bending backwards at the arch of the lower back? Does any pressure or tension in your lower back increase as you rock back? Keep sensing this tension as you watch the movement of your upper torso and, with patience, a clear pattern will emerge.

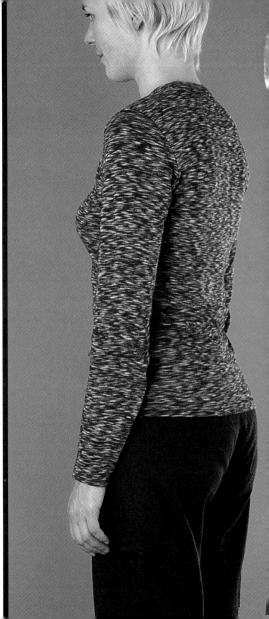

Pelvis and leg movements

Now watch the movement of your pelvis during this rocking movement of the torso. When your upper torso bends back from the lower back, which direction is your pelvis pushed in? Does it arch back and increase the inward curve of the lower back? Does the whole pelvis move forwards to counteract the backwards movement of the upper torso? If you look carefully you might notice that both happen.

Your pelvis most probably arches backwards and up, leading to an increased curve in your lower back. This concave curve in your lower back is also a result of your rib cage and your upper torso bending back, with your lower back as the pivot for this movement. Together these two actions lead to an increased inward curve in your lower back and to greater tension and potential for pain.

As it arches back and up, your pelvis can be moved forwards in space by the forward movement of your legs at the ankle joint, rather like bringing your weight forward on to the front of your foot. However, your weight doesn't come forward because, to counteract this, you then lock your knees back.

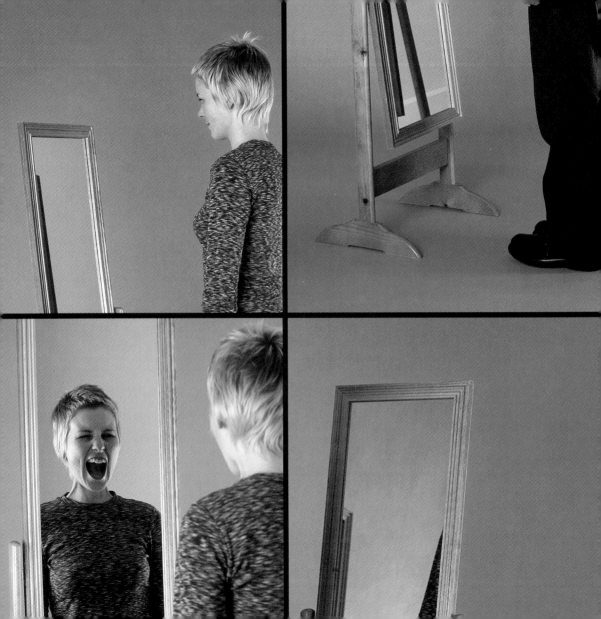

Analysing yourself

Spend time analysing the shortening in your body by observing and sensing your own co-ordination. Check out exactly what you do. Remember, we are not talking about something that is fixed – it is a continuous, subtle activity. Tension is an activity of little movements that can be watched. It is an exquisitely subtle inner dance. Be patient, and keep going back and observing your co-ordination until your pattern is clear to you. This will take some considerable time. Once you are fully aware of what backwards, down and shortening mean for you, you are ready to experiment with their antidotes, which are forwards, up and lengthening.

Experiencing forwards

Stand in front of your mirrors and take time to become sensitive to your body, repeating your whole previous analysis of your stance, co-ordination and tension. Monitor all your movements, keep checking the relationships between them, and become aware of all the specifics of your co-ordination. Remember that you are not trying to learn anything new, but are unlearning what you already do. Without this understanding you are merely imposing one set of habits upon another.

Start by very subtly thinking of releasing your head (not your neck) forwards as you feel its backward pull. The subtle release forwards of the head only happens as you can sense the tightening of it going back. As you feel a slight increase of tension in the back of your neck, think of releasing your neck muscles in a way that allows your head to tilt forwards. Check that you aren't tightening under the chin and throat: this will happen if you tighten muscles to pull your head forwards, rather than lengthening the muscles that pulled it back.

Continue releasing your head forwards by letting the muscles of the neck be free. Each time there will be a little more to release. Paradoxically, the more you release the head forwards, the more easily you can feel it tightening back. It will never be quite the same twice in a row and that is why it is so essential to release your head forwards in relation to the feeling of it going back.

You may start to feel a subtle improvement in the pattern of movement throughout your whole body. Your breathing may become less constricted, the pressure on your lower back less, the whole effort of standing easier. If you don't feel that, go back and watch more carefully, working until you can sense that this tiny release of your head forwards affects the whole pattern of movement. Persistence will pay off, impatience will not.

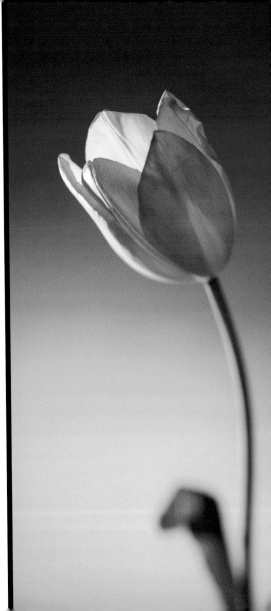

Experiencing forwards and up

Forwards refers to the movement of your head and only your head. It does not mean you want your neck to go down. All 'head forwards' means is preventing your head from going back.

Up refers to your neck and whole body. While there are more than a hundred muscles that can pull your neck down, it is only by releasing those muscles that you can achieve neck up.

As you are aware of tilting your head forwards, become aware of the forward, downward pressure that results in the neck down movement. Can you relieve that pressure by decreasing the tension in your neck by taking your neck up? It's easy to make the neck look like it goes up if you increase tension, but the point here is to experiment until you are able to think it up in a way that reduces the feeling of strain. The key is to ensure that your head continues in its head forwards orientation as you experiment with releasing your neck up.

In your eagerness to succeed, it will be easy to delude yourself that there isn't an increase of tension in your neck. This requirement of increased ease and freedom in your neck is the guiding principle of your experiment, and you must be able to achieve even a little of this before carrying on any further. That could take you months to figure out. Alternatively, it could happen instantly. Everyone is different.

Until this point, whatever you thought was forwards and up probably wasn't forwards and up. In fact, forwards and up is never going to feel the same twice in a row if you're doing these experiments correctly.

Experiencing forwards and up and lengthening

If you find that you are starting to fall backwards as you experience forwards and up, you are ready to move on. For the majority of people (there are exceptions) the reason you fall backwards is because your upper torso is bending back. It did that to counteract the falling forwards of your neck, but since your neck is not doing that anymore, your torso is out of line, so you start to fall backwards instead.

So now, as you counteract the tightening of your head and neck by allowing them to release head forwards and neck up, you also allow your whole torso to move forwards through space. Using mirrors becomes indispensable at this point, as when you succeed (and success means reduced tension, easier breathing, a sense of tallness, lightness and ease), you will feel as though you are leaning forwards or that your bottom is sticking out at the back. But if you look carefully in the mirror you should see that actually you have straightened up. If you are leaning forwards then you need to go back and find the moment where you went wrong.

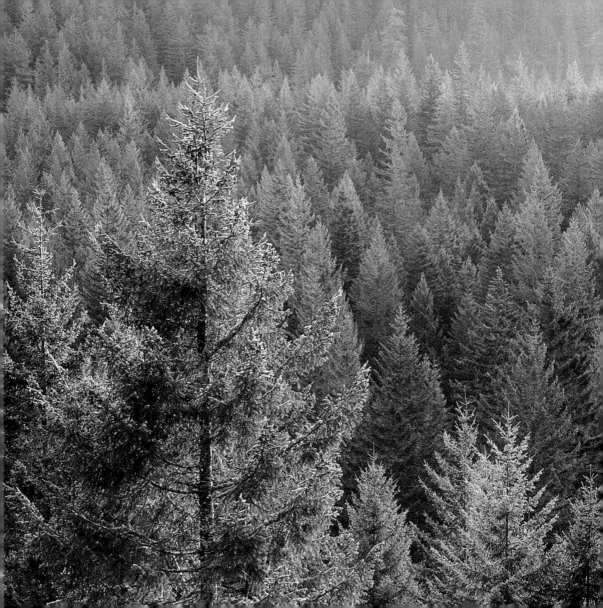

Integration

The way to allow your upper torso to ease forwards is by directing your head forwards while lengthening up, but the way for your head to go forwards is by lengthening up, which is caused by easing your upper torso forwards! It is easy to activate the second direction while you are also activating the first, but it is difficult to realize either unless you activate both together.

All the directions you give yourself in Alexander work act like this: each one points itself towards the next one so that the sum is greater than the parts. They integrate when they occur together, one after the other. You do the first direction to cause the second direction, then you immediately project the first and the second directions in order to cause the third and so on.

Alexander adopted the phrase 'thinking in activity' for this purpose of projecting a number of different directions together in their sequence. In practice this means that as you explore sensations in your body you expand your attention to become more inclusive. For example, as you bring an awareness to your torso, continue with your awareness of your head and neck. Practise understanding the links, the continuity between the different areas. How does one connect into the next?

By thinking in activity and collecting together the awareness of several areas all together, one after the other, there is a greater chance that you will discover a pattern of holding of which you had previously been unaware. By understanding the holistic operation of your co-ordination, you have a better chance of unmasking the patterns that create unnecessary tension.

Alexander spent many, many years coming to understand how all the directions work together but you can experience this in the space of a few minutes under the skilful guidance of a teacher's hands. In these experiments, if you fail to link the directions together it won't work. The good news is that by combining directions you can generate powerful experiences of release. The small releases you had to begin with are going to increase in their magnitude until it all begins to feel quite magnificent and magical.

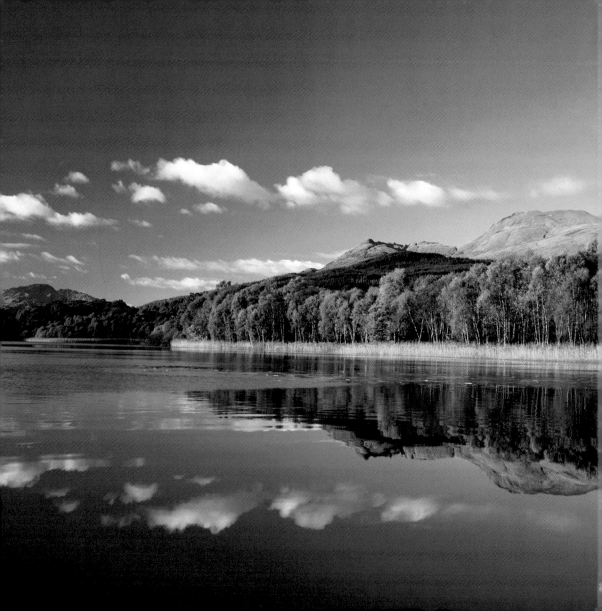

What Next?

Working through all the procedures and experiments described here is only the beginning. The more elements you combine, the greater the complexity.

Alexander work is a journey, an exploration into a whole new field of enquiry, and the more you investigate, the more the results encourage you to continue. As Alexander once so aptly put it: 'There is so much to be seen when one reaches the point of being able to see, and the experience makes the meat it feeds upon.'

Useful Addresses and Websites

International

Alexander Technique International (ATI)
Head Office:
1692 Massachusetts Ave, 3rd floor
Cambridge, MA 02138 USA
Tollfree: +1 888-668-8996
(Canada and USA only)
Tel: +1 617-497-2242
Fax: +1 617-497-2615
E-mail: usa@ati-net.com

Australia

Australian Society of Teachers of the
Alexander Technique (AUSTAT)
PO Box 716
Darlinghurst, NSW, 2010
Freecall: 1800 339 571
Email: Austat@alextech.net

United Kingdom

Society of Teachers of the Alexander
Technique (STAT)
129 Camden Mews, London 9AH
Tel: +44 020 7284 3338 Email:
Info@stat.org.uk

United States

American Society of Teachers of the
Alexander Technique (AmSAT)
P.O. Box 60008, Florence, MA 01062
Tel: (800) 473-0620 / 413-584-2359
Email: Amsat@alextech.net

Canada

Canadian Society of Teachers of the
Alexander Technique (CanSTAT)
465 Wilson Avenue
Toronto
Ontario M3H IT9
Tel: (877) 598 8879

Ireland

Alexander Technique International
Kirkullen Lodge
Tooreeny
Moycullen
Co. Galway
Tel: (0) 91 555 800

South Africa

South African Society of Teachers of the
Alexander Technique (SASAT)
17 Ash Street
Observatory 7925
Tel: 027 447 9436

Websites

www.directionjournal.com
Large collection of high quality articles on an amazing array of Alexander-related topics.

www.alexandertechnique.net
First stop web site with an international database of teachers, training schools and societies.

www.alexandertechnique.com
Introductory site with general information for beginners.

www.alexandertech.com
American Society (AmSAT) website. Links to other affiliated national societies.

www.alexandertechnique.org.au
Australian Society (AUSTAT) website. Contact details of all teacher members.

www.ati-net.com
Alexander Technique International website. Articles and links to all national offices.

www.stat.org.uk
UK Society of Teachers of the Alexander Technique (STAT) website. Contact details of all teacher members; information on books, links to other affiliated national societies.